DK The British Medical Association

FAMILY DOCTOR GUIDE *to*

ALLERGIES & HAY FEVER

PROFESSOR ROBERT DAVIES

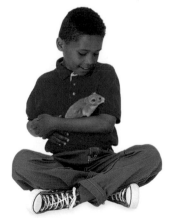

MEDICAL EDITOR
DR. TONY SMITH

DORLING KINDERSLEY
LONDON • NEW YORK • SYDNEY • MOSCOW
www.dk.com

IMPORTANT

This book is not designed as a substitute for personal medical advice but as a supplement to that advice for the patient who wishes to understand more about his/her condition.

Before taking any form of treatment **YOU SHOULD ALWAYS CONSULT YOUR MEDICAL PRACTITIONER.**

In particular (without limit) you should note that advances in medical science occur rapidly, and some of the information contained in this book about drugs and treatment may very soon be out of date.

PLEASE NOTE

The author regrets that he cannot enter into any correspondence with readers.

A DORLING KINDERSLEY BOOK
www.dk.com

Senior Editor Mary Lindsay
Senior Designer Sarah Hall
Production Assistant Elizabeth Cherry

Managing Editor Stephanie Jackson
Managing Art Editor Nigel Duffield

Produced for Dorling Kindersley Limited by
Design Revolution, Queens Park Villa,
30 West Drive, Brighton, East Sussex BN2 2GE
Editorial Director Ian Whitelaw
Art Director Fiona Roberts
Editor Julie Whitaker
Designer Vanessa Good

Published in Great Britain in 1999 by
Dorling Kindersley Limited,
9 Henrietta Street, London WC2E 8PS

2 4 6 8 10 9 7 5 3 1

A CIP catalogue record for this book is available from the British Library

ISBN 07513 0675 4

Reproduced by Colourscan, Singapore
Printed in Hong Kong by Wing King Tong

Contents

What is an allergy?

Hay fever, asthma and other allergies have become much more common over the last hundred years and, are now an important cause of illness, especially in children and young adults.

This book explains how allergies develop, describes the common symptoms and gives detailed practical advice on how sufferers can recognise their own individual causes, and so avoid them whenever possible.

It explains the medical treatments that are currently available, including useful self-help measures for emergencies.

THE BODY'S RESPONSE
The symptoms of an allergic reaction vary from person to person, but often include violent attacks of sneezing and watery eyes.

ALTERED REACTIONS

Allergy is a word widely used to describe anything from an attack of sneezing and runny eyes on a warm sunny day, to an itchy red rash and wheezing after stroking the family pet, or to swelling of the lips and tongue and vomiting after eating a peanut. Allergy simply means an altered reaction, and is best thought of as the inappropriate and harmful response of the body's defence mechanism to substances that are normally harmless.

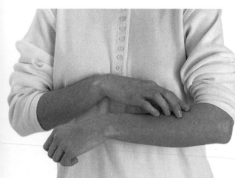

A SKIN REACTION
Many allergy sufferers experience an uncomfortable, itchy skin rash after contact with a particular substance.

The most common allergies are:

- Hay fever and itchy eyes (allergic conjunctivitis)
  - Asthma
  - Itchy skin rashes
- Food allergies
- Allergy to wasp and bee stings.

Allergic reactions to medicine and drugs such as antibiotics and local anaesthetics are less common, but many asthma and hay fever sufferers find that taking aspirin and other similar drugs make their symptoms worse.

Many people who suffer a lot from stomachache, diarrhoea and constipation, as well as those experiencing severe headaches, hyperactivity or lassitude often put their problems down to food, although this is difficult to classify as true allergy; these reactions are best described as intolerances.

While you may get hay fever, asthma or itchy skin rashes (contact dermatitis) through breathing in or touching reactive chemicals at work, the environment in certain offices can cause what is known as 'sick building syndrome'. This is most likely in air-conditioned buildings that have artificial lighting, wall-to-wall carpet and windows that cannot be opened. Symptoms of 'sick-building syndrome' include itchy eyes, dry throat and feelings of lassitude.

A number of people believe that they develop symptoms and feel unwell on contact with many of the chemicals used in everyday life, such as washing powders, bleaches and aerosol cleaning sprays, and they find it difficult to exist outside highly controlled environments free of such materials. This is known as multiple chemical sensitivity and, while it is real enough to the sufferers, it is difficult to explain scientifically, and is at present not known to be a manifestation of allergy.

════ HOW COMMON IS ALLERGY? ════

There is no doubt that allergies are on the increase, although some are more common than others.

- One in three people will suffer from an allergy at some time in their lives.
- One person in five suffers from hay fever. It was almost unknown until the 20th century and in the same way as allergies in general, hay fever appears to be a disease of prosperous countries.
- One in five schoolchildren is thought to be affected by asthma.
- One in six children has skin conditions associated with allergy, particularly eczema.
- One in 20 people suffers the itchy raised rash known as urticaria.
- Food allergies, particularly to peanuts, seem to be increasing at a dramatic rate although, fortunately, they are still relatively uncommon.
- A large local reaction to bee and wasp stings occurs in 10 per cent of the population.

WHY IS ALLERGY INCREASING?

Allergies run in families. There are two key factors that determine whether you will develop an allergic disease. The first is your genetic make-up. The allergy gene controlling production of the allergy antibody immunoglobulin E (IgE), and the inflammation that leads to allergic reactions, is positioned on the fifth of the 46 chromosomes in your DNA. The second factor is your exposure to the allergen – the substance that causes the reaction. In most of the common allergies, you need to have encountered the allergen early in life.

The rapid increase in allergies cannot be put down to a change in genetic make-up since this would take several generations, so it must be a result of changes in the environment and in lifestyle. An example of this process can be seen in the rapid increase in allergic diseases that is being detected in eastern European countries that are rapidly assuming the western (European) way of life. The kind of changes that are important include a decrease in worm infestation, fewer childhood infections and dramatic changes in living conditions in the home. The allergy mechanism is most effective at preventing worms in the gut from entering the body. If this mechanism is no longer required to deal with worm infestation, it is possible that it will now direct its effects against less harmful intruders, such as pollen grains, for example. Younger children in large families suffer much less from allergy than their older brothers and sisters. This is thought to be related to the more frequent viral infections readily passed from one child to another in large families.

First-born children, in whom allergies are more common, escape these infections, which are thought to tilt the reactions of the immune system away from producing the allergy antibody. A general decrease in family size leads to a higher proportion of children being affected by allergic diseases.

THE FIRST-BORN CHILD
The eldest child in a family is more likely to suffer from an allergy than younger siblings. The eldest has less exposure to viral infections and are therefore more likely to produce allergy antibodies.

MODERN FACTORS

Studies from Sweden, Germany and Japan have shown urban and rural differences in the frequency of the common allergic diseases. This suggests that modern-day pollution may be an important factor in the increase in allergic disorders. The most important components of this pollution are thought to be high levels of the nitrogen dioxide (NO_2) and, in particular, small particles present in the air in large numbers, largely due to emissions from diesel engines. Japanese and German studies have shown that allergies are more common in adults and children who live within 100 metres of busy roads, compared with those living in less polluted parts of cities.

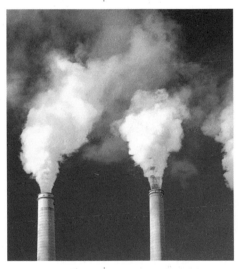

THE POLLUTED AIR
Emissions from factories and exhaust fumes are a major source of pollution. Poor air quality is thought to exacerbate hay fever and asthma.

These results have not been confirmed in the UK, possibly due to the fact that a major pollutant, ozone, can be found at high levels in the countryside, much of it being carried across from continental Europe. High levels of small particulates are also found in the air in rural communities. Although the debate continues about the importance of air pollution in increasing allergies, there is no doubt that those people suffering from asthma and hay fever can be made worse on days of high pollution.

Indoor pollution is the major contributor to the epidemic of allergies seen today. The need to conserve energy, important as it is, has led to a transformation in the indoor condition in houses. Coal fires and lack of double glazing and insulation meant that houses in the

What Causes Allergy?

The following factors are the most common allergens. They commonly act as allergy triggers in susceptible individuals, and some people are allergic to several of these.

HOUSE DUST MITE	The house dust mite, and particularly its droppings (faeces), is the most common cause of allergy, affecting up to 90 per cent of allergy sufferers.
GRASS POLLEN	Grass pollen causes a reaction in some 70 per cent of allergy sufferers, and the amount in the air will increase if more farmland is set aside for ungrazed meadows.
PETS	Pets are the next most important cause of allergic symptoms, with 40 per cent of asthmatic children sensitised to the allergens of cats or dogs.
TREES	Trees are a common cause of early springtime hay fever. Global warming has meant that new plants, for example *Parietaria judaiica*, or wall pellitory, previously confined to continental Europe, are now appearing in southern England. As warming increases, birch pollen will become more of a problem, and even pollen from olive trees may be blown from Europe to the UK, as olive trees extend northwards from the Mediterranean.
MOULDS	Moulds can trigger hay fever in the autumn, while spores from moulds such as *Aspergillus fumigatus* and *Alternaria* are very common in the atmosphere and can cause very severe attacks of asthma.
FOOD ALLERGIES	Milk, egg, fish and now peanuts are major causes of food allergies, and colourings and preservatives can trigger attacks.

past were draughty, with up to seven changes of the air in a room in every hour. Now that we have fewer chimneys, more effective insulation, double-glazing and central heating, air exchanges in the rooms of modern houses may be less than one per hour. As a result, humidity levels are high.

In addition, most homes have more soft furnishings and fitted carpets, together creating an ideal environment for the house dust mite and the retention of allergens from pets, fumes from unventilated gas cookers, cigarette smoke and the fumes and vapours from household chemicals and sprays. This mixture of allergens and irritants in the unventilated home environment is likely to be the major cause of the rapid increase in allergic diseases.

INDOOR POLLUTION
Smoking and cooking produce irritating fumes that can remain trapped indoors, especially in modern homes, which are far less well ventilated than older houses.

EARLY EXPOSURE

The allergic reaction begins early in life in people who are genetically predisposed. Exposure to both indoor and outdoor allergens, such as the house dust mite and pets, and pollens and moulds in a baby's first year leads to the production of the allergy antibody immunoglobulin E or IgE. The amount of exposure at this time is critical. A child who is exposed to high levels of house dust mite allergen in the first year of life is statistically more likely to develop asthma in childhood and in the teens.

Similarly, children born during the pollen season are more likely to develop hay fever. IgE antibody fixes to specialised cells called mast cells, which contain large amounts of histamine and other powerful chemicals called leukotrienes, which can dilate blood vessels and constrict the smooth muscle encircling the airways of the lung.

13

Mast Cells at Work

In susceptible individuals, who have produced antibodies as the result of exposure to allergens, contact with an allergen causes the mast cells to release histamine and other chemicals, producing allergic symptoms.

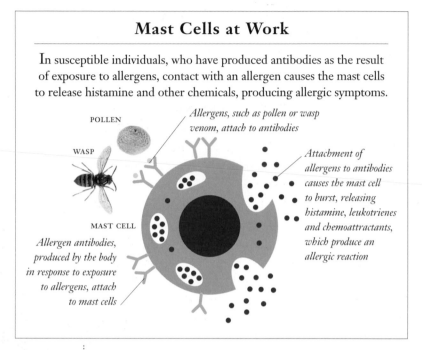

POLLEN

Allergens, such as pollen or wasp venom, attach to antibodies

WASP

Attachment of allergens to antibodies causes the mast cell to burst, releasing histamine, leukotrienes and chemoattractants, which produce an allergic reaction

MAST CELL

Allergen antibodies, produced by the body in response to exposure to allergens, attach to mast cells

They also attract other specialised cells, particularly the white blood cells known as eosinophils, which can cause inflammation and damage.

Histamine and the leukotrienes cause itching and sneezing, together with swelling in the skin, in the tubes of the lungs (the airways) and in the lining of the nose. This results in itchy red lumps in the skin, asthma and nasal blockage. The inflammation induced by the attraction of eosinophils leads to increased sensitivity of the lining of the nose and lung, and the development of chronic symptoms. Other cells, called lymphocytes, also play a key role in the persistent inflammation that characterises eczema and contact dermatitis in particular, but which is also a feature of hay fever and asthma.

HOW ALLERGY IS DIAGNOSED

There are a number of possible tests that can detect whether your symptoms are due to an allergy and can identify the allergen(s) responsible.

SKIN PRICK TESTING

Mast cells to which the allergy antibody, IgE, has attached are found throughout the skin and in the lining of the nose, the mouth, the tongue, the lung airways and throughout the intestines. Your skin can be used as a test site to simulate what is happening in other parts of your body. A tiny prick is made into your skin with a needle or lancet through a drop of the allergen. Usually, the test will be done on the skin on your forearm or back. If the allergen provokes a release of histamine, you will develop a red, itchy reaction within a few minutes. It then swells with a blister-like weal in the centre, reaching its maximum in about 20 minutes and fading within a few hours. The size of the weal correlates roughly with the level of your allergy to that particular allergen. The prick test introduces such a tiny amount of allergen into the skin that testing is quite safe and can be carried out on almost any age group. Twenty to thirty allergens can be tested at the same time.

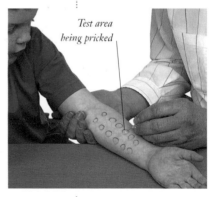

Test area being pricked

TESTING FOR ALLERGIES
The doctor places drops of suspected allergens on the skin, and pricks the skin through each drop with a small needle or lancet. An allergic reaction produces a red, itchy weal.

It takes some time for the mast cells throughout the body to become coated with IgE antibody, so skin tests may be negative in a child under the age of three, even though he or she is actually allergic to the allergen. Even when you have a positive test to a particular allergen, you may not get any symptoms when you come into contact with it because the body has mechanisms, at present ill-understood, which can dampen down the reaction to inhaled allergens. When positive skin tests correlate with symptoms, you can be certain that they are caused by an allergy to that particular allergen.

SKIN PATCH TESTS

In this test, solutions of common allergens causing contact dermatitis – such as ingredients of cosmetics, nickel or preservatives – are placed on the skin of your back and left under a special dressing for three days. If you develop an itchy, red raised patch, it means the result is positive. Taken in conjunction with a history of skin symptoms these tests have a high level of accuracy.

BLOOD TESTS (CAP-RAST)

Blood tests (known as CAP-RAST) are increasingly used to test for the presence of IgE antibody in the blood. Unlike skin tests, these tests can accurately measure the precise amount of the allergy antibody present in blood, and the results are commonly graded on a scale of zero to six.

When no or very little antibody (0 or 1) is found, you are unlikely to have any allergic disease, but moderate or high levels (2 and above) are associated with allergic disease. As with skin testing, 20 or 30 allergens can be tested in one blood sample.

These blood tests are particularly useful if you are taking an antihistamine to control your allergy, as this would block skin test reactions, or if you have widespread eczema, making skin prick or skin patch testing extremely difficult.

OTHER TESTS

A number of other tests for allergy are available. These include the neutralisation/provocation test (the Miller technique); cytotoxic tests of blood cells; hair analysis; Vega testing; applied kinesiology; and the auricular cardiac reflex method. The rationale for these tests is poorly understood and the results do not often match those produced by skin prick testing, patch testing or CAP-RAST testing. At the present time these tests are not recommended.

DRUGS FOR ALLERGIES

The most important factor in treating allergy is identifying the allergen that causes your symptoms, and avoiding contact with it as far as possible. However, there are several different groups of medicines that, when properly used, can, not only relieve symptoms, but can also reduce the ongoing inflammation of tissues that is caused by chronic allergies.

DECONGESTANTS

Decongestant nasal drops or sprays such as ephedrine and xylometazoline (Otrivine or Sudafed) act by constricting the blood vessels supplying the lining of the nose, causing shrinking of the nasal tissue and relief of nasal obstruction.

These drugs act rapidly and are very effective, but you should not use them for long periods at a time because shutting off the blood supply by constricting the blood vessels in this way can cause tissue damage and worsening of your symptoms.

DECONGESTANT SPRAYS
These drugs are inhaled through the nose. They relieve congestion, but they should not be used for prolonged periods.

BRONCHODILATORS

Bronchodilator drugs work by relaxing the constricted smooth muscle that is narrowing the airways of the lungs of people with asthma.

Spacer device

Inhaler

They act quickly and are very effective for people with mild asthma who only get occasional attacks of wheezing after contact with an allergen or after exercise. However, you should not rely on them if your asthma is more severe, since they do not treat the ongoing chronic inflammation. To stop this getting worse, you will also need treatment with inhaled anti-allergic drugs such as sodium cromoglycate (Intal), nedocromil sodium (Tilade) or steroids.

EASIER BREATHING
Bronchodilators provide rapid and effective relief for mild asthma. Children may benefit from using a spacer device.

EMOLLIENTS

Emollients soothe and moisturise the skin and are the basic treatment for all itchy, scaling skin disorders.

Several different types of emollient are available, such as Aqueous cream, Diprobase and E45. Although there is little difference between them, you may find that one product suits you better than the others. Most people prefer to use creams, which work into the skin, rather than ointments, which are greasy, and you may also be advised to add emollients to your bath water. Some people may develop an allergy to the preservatives contained in most emollients, however.

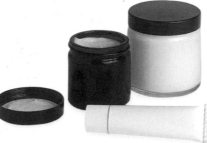

SOOTHING THE SKIN
Literally meaning 'softeners', emollients have a soothing and moisturising effect. They are used to treat dry, itchy or scaly conditions, including allergies.

ANTIHISTAMINES

Antihistamines were first discovered over 50 years ago, and are the mainstay of allergy treatment. In the last decade, several new and significantly different antihistamine preparations have become available – these are the so-called 'second generation antihistamines'.

Like 'first generation' antihistamines, these compounds (see p.35) block the action of histamine released from mast cells and are very effective in the treatment of itching and sneezing. However, they have considerable advantages over the older first generation antihistamines, such as chlorpheniramine (Piriton).

Second generation antihistamines have the advantage of not crossing into the brain, so they do not make you feel drowsy. This is a major plus point, because it means that taking the drug does not interfere with your ability to carry out complex tasks such as driving or operating machinery. They are also less likely to make your mouth feel dry.

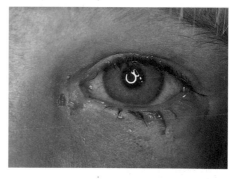

ANTI-ALLERGIC DRUGS

The group of anti-allergic drugs (also known as mast cell stabilisers), which includes sodium cromoglycate and nedocromil sodium, remains unique in that these drugs work by preventing the mast cells and eosinophils from releasing histamine and the other complex chemicals that cause inflammation.

ALLERGIC CONJUNCTIVITIS
Anti-allergic drugs are very good for treating conditions such as allergic conjunctivitis, a condition that affects the eyes. They are often used for long-term conditions, as they have few side-effects.

They have to be taken before you come into contact with the allergen – which means taking them regularly. Their remarkable lack of side-effects makes them very suitable for the treatment of allergic conditions, particularly allergic conjunctivitis, hay fever and

Drugs Used in the Treatment of Allergies

Once an allergy has been diagnosed, it is possible to treat it with drugs. There are many different types of drugs available. The following are some of the most commonly used.

DECONGESTANTS	Nasal spray; fast-acting drugs used to relieve nasal congestion.
BRONCHODILATORS	Inhaler; used to relax the smooth bronchial muscle, allowing air to move freely through the airways.
EMOLLIENTS	Ointment/cream; used to soothe patches of inflamed skin.
ANTIHISTAMINES	Tablets or syrup; they block the inflammatory effects of histamine.
ANTI-ALLERGIC DRUGS	Inhaler or ointment/cream; work by preventing the release of histamine and other inflammatory chemicals.
CORTICOSTEROIDS	Inhaler or ointment/cream; powerful drugs used to relieve inflammation in the air passages or on the skin.

asthma, especially in children who need long-term therapy when there is concern about the side-effects of other groups of drugs.

CORTICOSTEROIDS

Corticosteroids are powerful and effective anti-allergic and anti-inflammatory drugs. Although they do not block the release of histamine and other complex chemicals from mast cells, they are very effective at relieving the inflammation that characterises chronic skin conditions associated with allergy, prolonged and severe hay fever (especially with a blocked nose) and moderately severe and chronic asthma. They operate at the level of the genes within the cells, preventing them from making important chemical messengers called cytokines, which influence the body's immune system at a very fundamental level.

While this group of compounds undoubtedly works well, there is concern about the side-effects (such as acne, facial reddening, fluid retention, muscle weakness and peptic ulcer), which almost inevitably follow when you take any of them in tablet form.

For this reason, corticosteroids have been formulated as nasal sprays for hay fever, inhalers for asthma and creams for the treatment of skin allergies. In addition, the newer synthetic corticosteroids, such as budesonide (Pulmicort) and fluticasone propionate (Flixotide), are very effective on the surface of the lungs, nose or skin, but are not absorbed well into the bloodstream. The small amount that is absorbed is rapidly removed again by the liver.

While we know that regular and prolonged use of steroid creams can lead to thinning and alterations in pigmentation of the skin, it is, as yet, not known fully whether the nasal and inhaled steroids have significant side-effects. There are concerns that the rate of growth in children may be reduced after prolonged and heavy usage of inhaled steroids. In addition, there have been instances of people bruising more easily, and there is also the possibility that cataracts could develop in a person's eyes following use of these drugs.

Corticosteroids remain the most effective treatment for allergies, but they are most suitable for those people who have more severe disease that has not responded to other medicines.

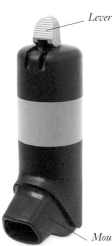

Lever

Mouthpiece

CORTICOSTEROIDS
These drugs are generally inhaled (using a device as illustrated), taken as a nasal spray or used in a cream. They are powerful anti-inflammatory agents.

KEY POINTS

- Allergies have become much more common in the last hundred years.
- Symptoms are caused by an overreaction of the body's immune system to a harmless substance.
- Allergies often run in families.
- Several allergy triggers have been identified. These include house mite, grass pollen and pets.
- Doctors use a number of tests to diagnose allergy.
- There are several different types of drugs available to relieve symptoms and reduce inflammation.

Hay fever and itchy eyes

Attacks of sneezing, runny and blocked nose, together with itchy and watery eyes in summer was first called 'hay fever' in the middle of the 19th century. Although we still use the term, in fact fever is not a symptom of the disease, nor is it due to hay!

ITCHY EYES
Eye drops can relieve the discomfort of allergic conjunctivitis, a common symptom of hay fever that results in watery, itchy eyes.

A more accurate name for hay fever is 'seasonal allergic rhinitis', the main cause of which is allergy to pollen. The symptoms of hay fever, or allergic rhinitis, can occur all year round, when it is called perennial rhinitis, and the main allergens involved are those from the house dust mite and pets.

Hay fever is the most common truly allergic condition and has become much more common in recent years, now affecting one in five of the population. As you will know only too well if you are a sufferer, not just your nose is affected. One of the most troublesome symptoms is itchy eyes that water all the time, a

Physical Symptoms of Hay Fever

In hay fever, the allergic reaction to an airborne irritant has effects mainly in the head. Itchiness is a common symptom, and may occur in the eyes, nose, throat and ears. A runny nose and watery eyes are also common.

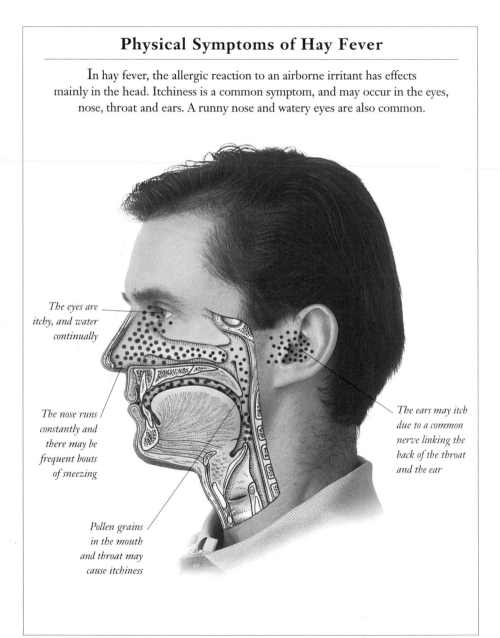

The eyes are itchy, and water continually

The nose runs constantly and there may be frequent bouts of sneezing

Pollen grains in the mouth and throat may cause itchiness

The ears may itch due to a common nerve linking the back of the throat and the ear

condition known as allergic conjunctivitis, and in up to a third of hay fever sufferers itching, red and running eyes are the major symptom. Moreover, 50 per cent of hay fever sufferers also have symptoms of asthma.

Hay fever is most common, and also at its most severe, in people in their teens, which causes particular problems because symptoms are at their worst in May, June and July, just when students have to take critical examinations.

HAY FEVER SYMPTOMS

Your mouth, ears and throat can all be itchy if you suffer from hay fever.

ITCHING AND SNEEZING

The most important role of your nose is to filter air and protect your lungs. Itching and sneezing result from the effects of histamine released into the tissues of your nose during the allergic reaction to pollen. Irritation of just a very small area of the nose can result in instantaneous and vigorous sneezing, typically in bouts of five to 20 sneezes at a time. Your mouth may itch as well, because pollen is swept from your nose into the back of your throat.

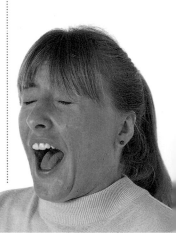

SNEEZING FITS
Irritation of the nasal lining can cause frequent and uncontrollable bouts of sneezing during an attack of hay fever.

Some people find their ears itch too, not through pollen landing in their ears, but as the result of the activation of a common nerve that links the back of the throat to the ear.

RUNNY NOSE

The nostrils are kept clear by secretion of a sticky fluid, mucus. However, when you have an allergic reaction to pollen, your nose can secrete up to an egg-cupful of clean, watery fluid every hour that spills out, so you are constantly sniffing and blowing your nose.

STUFFY, BLOCKED NOSE

You may be among the half of all hay fever sufferers who have to put up with a blocked nose, the most distressing of nasal symptoms. This is the result of the swelling of the nasal tissue, which is caused by the release of histamine and the leukotrienes from mast cells following interaction with pollen grains.

When your nose is completely blocked, you suffer from headaches, disturbed sleep and mouth breathing, which causes your throat and tongue to feel dry when you wake up in the morning. In severe cases, you cannot smell or taste anything either.

SINUSITIS

The sinuses, which are air-filled cavities in the bones of the skull, open out into the nasal cavity. When the tissue in your nose swells, it obstructs the openings, and bacteria trapped in the sinuses can then multiply, causing an infection called sinusitis. Acute sinusitis is very painful and leads to a fever, and you feel really unwell.

ITCHY AND WATERING EYES

Pollen grains can easily get into your eyes, and there they can react with mast cells that are present in the conjunctiva, the membrane that covers the white part of the eye and lines the inside of the eyelid.

This membrane becomes itchy and inflamed, making your eye look red, and you produce more tears to wash away the offending substance, causing your eyes to run. Particles then accumulate in the inner corner of the eye, which you then rub to remove them. This, of course, irritates the tissues of the eye further, making your eye increasingly itchy.

General Effects of Hay Fever

People who have never had hay fever tend to underestimate the symptoms of this distressing allergy. According to a recent Gallup poll:

- 40 per cent of sufferers found that their work was affected by hay fever, mainly due to irritability and lack of concentration.
- 80 per cent of sufferers felt really unhappy, miserable, depressed, irritated or listless during the hay fever season.
- One in 10 said they had to take time off from work.
- Studies have shown that children with hay fever perform less well in school.
- 40 per cent of sufferers are self-conscious about the effects of hay fever on their appearance, causing restriction in their social lives.
- 25 per cent of drivers who suffer from hay fever have said that their ability to drive was affected, and that it was unsafe to drive when they had hay fever symptoms, which is obviously a significant finding.

PERENNIAL ALLERGIC RHINITIS

This condition produces symptoms all year round. Although the major allergens are the house dust mite and pets, symptoms are often worse in the summer time due to additional allergy to pollen.

A blocked, stuffy nose is a more frequent symptom of perennial compared to seasonal rhinitis, although allergic conjunctivitis is less common. Children with persistent year-round symptoms often have bags under their eyes. Many children wipe their noses with the palms of their hands, pushing the tip of the nose upwards and causing the development of a crease across the nose.

IRRITANTS: HAY FEVER

Most sufferers first develop symptoms of hay fever when the density of pollen grains in the air reaches a figure of about 50 grains per cubic metre of air. However, as the season progresses and inflammation of the tissues builds up, fewer and fewer pollen grains are needed to trigger an attack in the very sensitive linings of the nose and eyes.

In addition, other irritants in the air, such as atmospheric pollution from traffic or industry, cigarette smoke, strong-smelling perfumes, household detergents and aerosols, can also trigger attacks, making your life as a hay fever sufferer even more unpleasant.

While you are not actually allergic to these irritant substances, you are very sensitive to their irritating effects because your eyes and the lining of your nose have become ultrasensitive due to their continuing allergic reaction to pollen.

INCIDENCE OF HAY FEVER
The incidence and severity of hay fever attacks vary throughout the year as the different allergens make their presence felt. Most sufferers respond to grass pollens, and these are at their highest levels in midsummer.

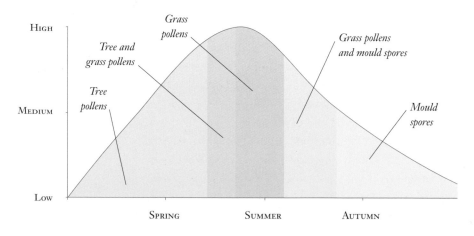

HIGH

Grass pollens

Tree and grass pollens

Tree pollens

Grass pollens and mould spores

MEDIUM

Mould spores

LOW

SPRING   SUMMER   AUTUMN

WHAT TRIGGERS HAY FEVER?

Hay fever sufferers are allergic to pollens present in the air. These come from wind-pollinated plants, by far the commonest of which are grasses, weeds and trees. Contrary to popular belief, it is rare for sufferers to be allergic to pollens from brightly coloured or scented plants, whose heavier, sticky pollens are transferred from plant to plant by insects.

GRASS POLLENS

Amongst the hundreds of species of grasses, only a relatively small number are sufficiently common and produce pollen in sufficiently large quantities to give high atmospheric pollen counts. Rye grass, extensively planted for grazing, produces less pollen than the traditional meadow grasses, including Timothy grass, cocksfoot, Yorkshire fog, sweet vernal grass and orchard grass.

As land is set aside from agricultural use, meadow grasses will once again dominate and consequently pollen counts are likely to rise.

There is extensive cross-reactivity between the grass species, so if you are allergic to one type, you may react to some extent to others.

The grass pollen season extends from mid-May to the end of July, peaking in late June and early July. The amount of pollen in the air varies from day to day and from hour to hour. Each grass species sheds its own pollen at a specific time of day. Although most species flower once daily in the early morning, two of the most prolific pollen producers, Yorkshire fog and sweet vernal grass, flower for a second time in the late afternoon.

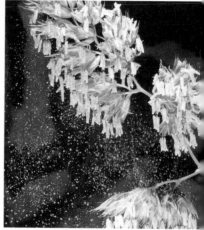

SHEDDING POLLEN
Since plant species shed their pollen at different times of day, the amount of pollen in the air in summer varies from hour to hour.

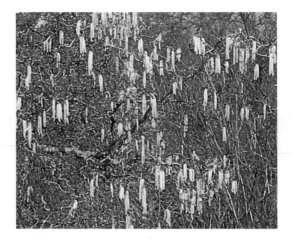

TOWN AND COUNTRY
Tree pollen is released in early spring. The planting of roadside trees, such as this hazel, has made tree pollen allergy as common in towns as it is in the countryside.

TREE POLLENS

The most common sources of tree pollens are the hazel, plane, oak, elm, ash and birch species, and their pollen is produced in the spring shortly after the leaves develop. The tree pollen season is shorter than that of grass pollen, lasting between four and six weeks from the end of March to the beginning of May.

WEED POLLENS

Unlike North America and the Mediterranean coastline, the climate of the UK does not favour the growth of ragweed, which is one of the most prolific pollen producers and a significant cause of hay fever in those regions. The pollens of various other weeds, however, can produce an allergic reaction.

Stinging nettle leaves are covered with hairs that inject histamine-releasing factors into the skin, causing the typical pain, itching and rash. Nettles flower in late summer and autumn, injecting pollen into the air as the sun shines on the curled young flowers. Fortunately, allergy to their pollens appears relatively uncommon.

However, a member of the same family, *Parietaria judaiica*, better known as wall pellitory, produces large amounts of highly allergenic pollen and is a major cause of hay fever symptoms across continental Europe. Unfortunately, this plant has now gained a foothold in southern England where it has begun to cause symptoms in the late summer and early autumn months.

OIL SEED RAPE

Over the last decade there has been a considerable increase in the commercial cultivation of the oil seed rape species. Pollination is partly by wind, and partly by insect. Although the bright yellow colour of the flower makes its presence very obvious, few people are truly allergic to its pollen.

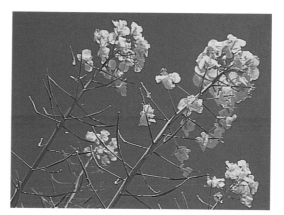

BLAMED FOR HAY FEVER
The sudden arrival of vivid fields of oil seed rape have made it a ready scapegoat for hay fever sufferers, but relatively few people are actually allergic to its pollen.

MOULDS

Moulds, a sub-division of the fungi, are very adaptable and may be found anywhere where there is moisture and oxygen. Typically they consist of long filaments that grow on the surface of organic materials such as compost heaps, rotten fruit or cheese.

● *Cladosporium herbarum* This mould produces a very large number of spores, and it is the most commonly encountered mould allergen. Particularly heavy spore concentrations occur between May and October, reaching up to 15,000 spores per cubic metre of air. The mould colonises foliage and plant matter, particularly grass, and the spores are a cause of hay fever during the summer months, especially when the grass is mown. If your symptoms do not coincide with the grass pollen count, allergy to *Cladosporium* may be the reason.

● *Alternaria alternata* This is another extremely common mould, found in soil compost and rotten wood, and it is a major cause of allergic disease in the USA. In this country, *Alternaria* causes rhinitis and asthma in the autumn, particularly during harvest time.

GLOBAL WARMING AND HAY FEVER

Some temperate areas of Europe, including southern England, have shown an increase in temperature of up to 0.5 degrees centigrade since 1970. If this trend continues, life will be even more unpleasant for hay fever sufferers. The hay fever season would extend, with grasses flowering earlier in the year and continuing into the late autumn. In addition, birch pollen would be produced earlier in the year, and some people could develop allergy to pollen from olive trees. Most worrying is the possibility that ragweed could establish itself in the UK. The pollen is potent, with fewer grains needed to produce attacks of hay fever. Ragweed is a prolific producer of pollens, leading to the severe hay fever experienced by many sufferers in the USA.

WEATHER AND TIME OF DAY

Grass flowers open early in the morning and pollen is scattered into the air. On fine, clear days, as the temperature rises, air carries the pollen up through the atmosphere, sometimes to the height of cumulus clouds. When these convection currents cease as the Earth's surface cools in the early evening, pollen grains fall in concentrated clouds. The peak concentration of pollen in country areas is around 5–6 p.m., while in urban areas, the peak is delayed by one to two hours. On calm nights, pollen from high in the atmosphere will gently settle out in the still air, resulting in a second peak after midnight. This pattern can be disrupted by rain in the morning, delaying the opening of the grass flowers and, if it persists, reducing pollen counts that day.

Daily estimates of the pollen counts, expressed as the average number of grains per cubic metre of air during a

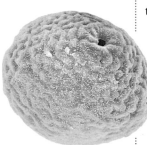

MICROSCOPIC CULPRIT
In the countryside, levels of pollen (seen here magnified many hundreds of times by an electron microscope) in the air normally reach a daily peak between 5 and 6 p.m.

24-hour period, are regularly reported during the spring and summer in newspapers and on television and radio weather broadcasts.

Thunderstorms can have a dramatic effect on the level of pollen allergen in the air. High humidity prior to a storm causes pollen grains to burst, liberating hundreds of small starch particles, which carry one of the major grass allergens. In cities, the allergens can attach to small carbon particles in the air, themselves the product of diesel engines. The starch granules, or allergens, attached to carbon particulates are readily inhaled, not only into the nose, but also into the airways of the lung.

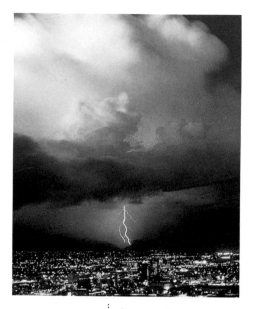

CHANGING POLLEN LEVELS
Levels of pollen allergen in the air may rise considerably during a thunderstorm, as the high humidity before a storm causes pollen grains to burst.

They were the cause of the remarkable outbreak of asthma in June 1994, which led to a dramatic increase in hospital admissions among hay fever sufferers who had never suffered from asthma previously. In addition, thunderstorms can lead to a dramatic increase in spore counts from a mould called *Didymella exitalis*, which is found on the leaves of ripening barley and wheat. The release of spores increases 25-fold after rainfall begins.

HOW IS HAY FEVER TREATED?

The treatment for hay fever, as with other allergies, is based on avoiding allergens. Since clouds of pollen grains are blown into urban areas, counts can be high even in the centre of a large city, and you cannot avoid them altogether. However, there are some steps you can take to reduce your exposure to pollen (see box on p.34).

Steps You Can Take to Reduce Exposure to Pollen

Whilst it may be physically impossible to avoid an airborne allergen such as pollen, you can reduce your exposure in the following ways.

- Avoid being outdoors in the early evening when pollen counts are at their highest.
- Try to stay indoors when the pollen count is high.
- Sleep with your bedroom windows closed to prevent pollen entering on still, calm nights.
- Wear sunglasses to help prevent pollen getting into your eyes.
- Get someone else to mow the lawn.
- When you are in the car, keep windows and doors shut; when buying a new car choose one with a pollen filter in the ventilation system.
- Take your holidays in coastal areas where sea breezes keep pollen inland.
- Take a shower and wash your hair in the evening to get rid of pollens.

DAIRY PRODUCTS
Some people find that cutting out dairy products from their diet helps to relieve the symptoms of hay fever, particularly a runny nose.

FOOD, DRUGS AND HAY FEVER

Food allergy rarely causes hay fever-like symptoms. However, some people find that cutting out dairy products from their diet alleviates nasal symptoms to some degree, particularly excessive nasal secretions. There is cross-reactivity between birch pollen and certain fruit allergens, particularly apples. About one in 20 people who have perennial rhinitis are sensitive to aspirin and other non-steroidal anti-inflammatory drugs such as ibuprofen (Nurofen), which can trigger symptoms and are associated with the development of nasal polyps.

DRUGS FOR HAY FEVER

The management of hay fever has been transformed by the fact that you can now buy virtually all the necessary treatments over the counter from the pharmacy without a prescription.

DECONGESTANTS

Oxymetazoline (Afrazine) and xylometazoline (Otrivine), taken as nasal drops or sprays, are the most commonly used decongestants.

They act rapidly, and help clear your blocked nose quickly and effectively. Their effect lasts for a relatively short time when they are used in this way. Ephedrine nasal drops are an alternative.

Topical decongestants also work very well, but you have to remember not to go on using them for more than 14 days. Using them for long periods can cause damage to the lining of the nose, making the blocked nose worse than ever once the effect of the drug has worn off. As a result, you are tempted to use them more and more often to try and clear your nose.

Decongestants are particularly useful in relieving nasal blockage before using an anti-inflammatory drug.

ANTIHISTAMINES

As you can now buy the modern, non-sedating, second-generation antihistamines from the pharmacy, you should always opt for one of these instead of the older, sedating antihistamines such as chlorpheniramine (Piriton) or clemastine (Tavegil).

Although these antihistamines are rarely associated with any drowsiness, you should take care when driving, and avoid drinking too much alcohol. Astemizole and

Over-the-Counter Antihistamines

These are all non-sedating, newer antihistamines that you can buy from the pharmacy without a prescription.

GENERIC NAME	BRAND NAME	DAILY DOSE
Cetirizine	Zirtek	10 mg once in the morning
Loratadine	Clarityn	10 mg once in the morning
Astemizole	Hismanal	10 mg once in the morning
Fexofenadine	Telfast	120 mg once in the morning

terfenadine have been associated with the development of serious rhythm disturbances of the heart in a very small proportion of hay fever sufferers. This is particularly the case in people taking the anti-fungal drug ketoconazole or the antibiotic erythromycin at the same time.

Since there is little to choose between the effectiveness of these drugs, it is best to avoid medication associated with these side-effects if possible. Fexofenadine is the active product of terfenadine after breakdown in the liver. Unlike terfenadine, it has no effect on the heart and is effective and safe and should be used instead of terfenadine. Loratidine, cetirizine and fexofenadine can be recommended as non-sedative and effective antihistamines.

These antihistamines can be sold for the treatment of hay fever in children over the age of 12. Your doctor can, however, prescribe these antihistamines for younger children. Loratadine can be prescribed for children over the age of two.

Not everyone responds to the same extent to each of the antihistamines, so you may need to try one or two before finding the preparation that suits you best.

There is another antihistamine, called acrivastine (Semprex), which is only available at the moment from your doctor. This needs to be taken three times a day.

Antihistamines can be sprayed directly into the nostrils,

The Aims of Treatment

The British Allergy Foundation has developed the following series of goals for the management of hay fever:

- The ideal is to allow sufferers to be free of the limitations caused by hay fever so that they can carry on with work or school as usual, and enjoy the spring and summer.
- Treatment should be aimed at reducing all symptoms of hay fever, including sneezing, runny nose and eyes and nasal blockage.
- In moderate and severe cases, treatment should be aimed at the underlying inflammation.
- Side-effects of treatment should not interfere with, or restrict, sufferers' daily activities or quality of life.
- Hay fever treatment should not prevent the sufferer from being able to drive or operate machinery.
- In order for sufferers to comply with therapy, dosage should be simple.
- There should be minimal risks of side-effects.
- There should be no interactions with any other medication that the sufferer is taking.

and one preparation, azelastine (Rhinolast), is available as a twice-daily nasal spray.

Whilst this preparation is very effective for relieving the nasal symptoms of rhinitis, it does not, unlike the antihistamines taken by mouth, have any effects on allergy symptoms affecting the eyes.

ANTI-ALLERGIC PREPARATIONS

These are the mainstay of treatment for more persistent rhinitis, and need to be taken on a regular basis. Sodium cromoglycate (Rhinacrom) prevents allergen interaction with the mast cell from releasing histamine and the leukotrienes, which is what causes your symptoms. It is useful in persistent rhinitis in both adults and children, and as a four per cent aqueous spray, can be used between two and four times a day.

You can buy it over the counter from the pharmacy in the form of Resiston 1, which is a combination of two per cent sodium cromoglycate spray together with xylometazoline as a decongestant.

Sodium cromoglycate is much more effective in treating allergic conjunctivitis, where it can be applied as eye drops up to four times a day or as an ointment to treat itchy eyelids.

You can buy these preparations from the pharmacy without a prescription, as Clariteyes or Opticrom. These eye drops do contain a preservative called benzalkonium, which can itself occasionally cause an allergic-type reaction.

When you are using these eyedrops or ointment, you should not wear soft contact lenses, as they could react with the preservative.

CORTICOSTEROIDS

These are the most effective treatment for moderate and severe hay fever, particularly when symptoms are persistent and include nasal blockage. They reduce inflammation in the lining of the nose and treat all symptoms effectively. For reasons that are not wholly understood, spraying these medicines into the nose also helps to relieve allergic conjunctivitis. The nasal sprays should be used regularly on a daily basis.

Corticosteroids can be given as tablets that act rapidly and very effectively and can be used over a period of up to 14 days. They give you complete freedom from

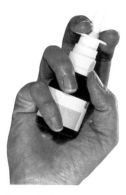

NASAL SPRAYS
Steroid nasal sprays are one of the most effective treatments for the symptoms of hay fever.

Steroid Nasal Sprays

Whilst all these preparations are very effective, Flixonase is probably the safest and most potent medicine for the treatment of hay fever, but it can only be obtained on prescription.

GENERIC NAME	BRAND NAME	DOSE	AVAILABLE OVER THE COUNTER?
Beclomethasone	Beconase Hay fever	2 sprays to each nostril morning and evening	Yes
Flunisolide	Syntaris	(as above)	Yes
Budesonide	Rhinocort	(as above)	No
Fluticasone	Flixonase	2 sprays to each nostril once daily in the morning	No
Triamcinolone	Nasacort	(as above)	No
Mometasone	Nasonex	(as above)	No

symptoms and are ideal for specific periods when you need to be on top form – for example, for key exams or a wedding. Long-lasting injections of corticosteroids are not recommended because of their side-effects.

HYPOSENSITISATION

Hyposensitisation, or specific allergen injection immuno-therapy treatment, involves injecting increasing amounts of purified grass pollen solution under your skin until your sensitivity to the allergen is reduced. To get the full benefit, you need to have injections monthly at the maximum dose over a period of 2–3 years.

This treatment can be very effective in severe hay fever that has not responded to anti-inflammatory treatment. Because of the dangers of severe reactions, which can include collapse (anaphylaxis), the injections can only be given in specialist hospital clinics where full resuscitation facilities are available. Those patients undergoing this treatment must be carefully observed for 60 minutes after each injection.

KEY POINTS

- The main symptoms of hay fever include a runny nose, itchy and watery eyes and sneezing.
- Hay fever sufferers are allergic to the pollens present in the air.
- Pollen levels fluctuate according to time of day and the weather.
- Antihistamine drugs, decongestants and corticosteroids help ease the symptoms of hay fever.

Asthma, cough and wheezing

Asthma is the only chronic disease in the developed world that is becoming more common. Studies of school children have shown that there has been a fourfold increase in the numbers suffering from asthma over the last 20 years.

Asthma is now the most common reason for children to be admitted to hospital, and in many areas is one of the leading causes of hospital admissions for adults as well. Tragically, asthma kills about 2,000 sufferers every year in the UK, many of them under the age of 35. Allergy is the most important cause of asthma, being implicated in 90 per cent of children and 50 per cent of adults with the disease.

WHAT IS ASTHMA?

The word asthma derives from Greek and literally means hard breathing, but its modern definition includes a description of its symptoms, the underlying mechanisms causing the disease, and its effect on the function and sensitivity of the lungs and their airways.

ASTHMA SYMPTOMS
During an asthma attack there is a feeling of tightness in the chest, and breathing is difficult.

41

The Respiratory System

The airways (trachea, bronchi and bronchioles) and airspaces within the lungs supply oxygen to and remove carbon dioxide from the body. Mucus is moved through the lungs by cilia (tiny hairs) on the airways' internal walls.

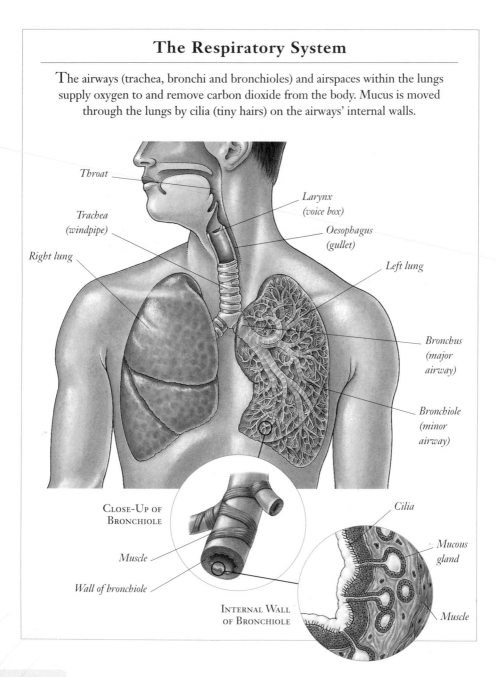

Throat

Larynx (voice box)

Trachea (windpipe)

Oesophagus (gullet)

Right lung

Left lung

Bronchus (major airway)

Bronchiole (minor airway)

CLOSE-UP OF BRONCHIOLE

Cilia

Muscle

Mucous gland

Wall of bronchiole

Muscle

INTERNAL WALL OF BRONCHIOLE

How Asthma Affects the Airways

During an asthma attack, the muscle walls of the airways (bronchi and bronchioles) contract, causing their internal diameter to narrow. Increased mucus secretion and inflammation of the airways' inner linings cause further narrowing.

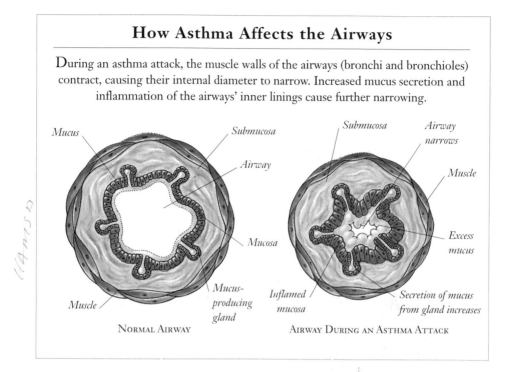

NORMAL AIRWAY

Mucus · *Submucosa* · *Airway* · *Mucosa* · *Mucus-producing gland* · *Muscle*

AIRWAY DURING AN ASTHMA ATTACK

Submucosa · *Airway narrows* · *Muscle* · *Excess mucus* · *Secretion of mucus from gland increases* · *Inflamed mucosa*

The symptoms of asthma are coughing, wheezing and shortness of breath, but the condition is characterised by a special type of inflammation of the lining of the airways of the lung. The key cells involved, as in other allergic diseases, are the mast cell and the eosinophil.

The effect of this inflammation on the lungs is to cause narrowing of the airways with a reduction in the amount of air that can be blown out of the lungs in a given time, and in the rate at which air can be expelled from the lungs. This obstruction to the flow of air out of the lungs can be completely, or partly, reversed by the inhalation of a bronchodilator. In addition, the inflammation of the airways causes them to be hypersensitive to many irritants such that the inhalation of cold air, pollution fumes, aerosols, household cleaning agents and disinfectants, and strong scents can trigger constriction of the irritated airways, giving rise to attacks of asthma.

WHAT ARE THE SYMPTOMS?

The symptoms of asthma include breathlessness, chest tightness, wheezing and coughing. The severity of the symptoms vary from day to day. During a severe attack, breathing may become very difficult.

SHORTNESS OF BREATH

Difficulty with breathing, a feeling of tightness in the chest and shortness of breath are the cardinal features of asthma. Their severity can vary from a short-lived feeling of breathlessness after exercise or after stroking the family pet, to disabling breathlessness, such that you cannot walk and do not have enough breath to complete a sentence. The hallmark of asthma is the variability in symptoms, so that on some days you feel fairly well, while at other times you are in need of urgent treatment.

A WHEEZY CHEST
Noisy wheezing is a frequent feature of asthma attacks. It is caused by air passing through swollen, blocked airways in the lungs.

WHEEZING

This whistling sound is the result of air being forced through swollen and partially obstructed airways in your lungs, causing whistling noises of different pitches.

Wheezy breathing is easily recognised, but it may not happen when the asthma is severe. This is because insufficient air is being blown out through the airways of the lungs to generate the noise.

COUGHING

A cough, especially at night, is a characteristic of asthma, as it is of many other lung diseases, particularly bronchitis induced by smoking or associated with a chest infection. It can be difficult for a doctor to diagnose whether a cough is actually the result of asthma rather than of some other lung condition.

Inflammation of the lung airways in babies and toddlers is frequently the result of viral infections. Infection with the respiratory syncytial virus gives rise to a troublesome and sometimes serious condition called bronchiolitis, which makes the lung airways (the bronchi) swell up. The young child then suffers wheezing and breathlessness, as well as fever. He or she will often have a cough for some time after one of these viral infections and, if there is a family history of asthma, this may be the first sign that the child is developing asthma. It is not surprising that young children are often treated with frequent courses of antibiotics before the correct diagnosis of asthma is made, and appropriate treatment with bronchodilators, anti-allergic and anti-inflammatory drugs started. Similarly, it can be very difficult to distinguish between bronchitis and asthma, particularly in adults who smoke and who are suffering prolonged episodes of coughing. It is important to make the correct diagnosis since bronchitis must be treated with antibiotics, while, on the other hand, an asthmatic cough will respond to appropriate anti-asthma treatment. Either way, it is extremely important to stop smoking.

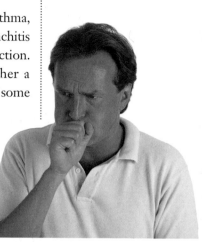

POSSIBLE SYMPTOM
Unexpected asthma may sometimes be the cause of a cough that occurs mainly at night.

INCREASED NIGHT-TIME SYMPTOMS

All the symptoms of asthma worsen during the night, disturbing your sleep and leaving you feeling tired the following day. The reason for this is that lung function in everybody is at its worst at four in the morning and at its best at four in the afternoon. This is due to the changes that occur in circulating levels of the hormone adrenaline, which are lowest in the middle of the night. Adrenaline helps to relax the muscles of the lung airways, keeping them open. Nerve impulses slow the heart and the activity of the intestines as the body shuts down during sleep, but at the same time cause minor narrowing of the airways of the lung. In addition, circulating levels of corticosteroids, which are so important in countering any inflammatory process in the body, are low in the early hours of the morning. While you will never notice these effects if you do not have asthma, their influence is greatly exaggerated in people who already have inflammation of the lung airways, making their symptoms and lung function worse at night.

ASTHMA AND EXERCISE
Exercise in wintry conditions can trigger an asthma attack, as cold, dry air affects the lining of the airways and produces a reaction.

EFFECT OF WINTER EXERCISE

Inhaling cold, dry air by breathing through your mouth when you are exercising leads to changes in the fluid lining the airways in the lung. This can trigger the release of histamine and other potent chemicals, including leukotrienes, from mast cells. This will lead to a brief attack of asthma that can last for

10–20 minutes and that can have a devastating effect on a child's ability to join in games in the playground and on the playing field, disrupting his or her social and physical development.

HOW IS IT DIAGNOSED?

In order to decide whether you have asthma, the doctors need to find out whether the degree of obstruction to the flow of air through your lung airways varies at different times. This task has been made much easier with the introduction of small airflow meters that you can use yourself to record the maximum rate at which you can blow air out of your lungs at different times of the day. The most widely used meter, available on prescription, is the Wright peak-flow meter. You blow as hard as possible through the meter and record the peak expiratory flow rate (PEFR). The maximum PEFR depends on your age, sex and height, and varies from approximately 600 litres per minute in a fit young man of average height to approximately 300 litres per minute in an older woman. Recordings in people with asthma show a reduced peak flow measured when they wake up compared to peak flows measured in the early evening. This pattern of variation is the same each day. A variation in the peak flow from morning to evening of 15 per cent or more confirms the diagnosis of asthma.

USING A PEAK-FLOW METER
You can measure the rate at which you exhale by using a peak-flow meter. Variations in the result can indicate asthma.

The peak-flow meter is also useful in monitoring the effects of treatment, which reduce the variation as well as improving the peak expiratory flow rate overall, since the more severe the asthma the lower the PEFR.

More sophisticated tests can be undertaken in special hospital lung function laboratories. These include the measurement of the amount of air that can be blown out of the lungs in one second (the forced expiratory volume in one second, or FEV1). This is an accurate test because the amount is reduced in asthma sufferers. An improvement in the FEV1 of 15 per cent or more after the inhalation of a bronchodilator confirms the diagnosis of asthma. Exercise or inhalation of solutions of histamine can be used to stress the lung, inducing a brief, short-lived fall in lung function in people with asthma.

WHAT ARE THE ALLERGENS?

It is important to identify the allergen that is causing your asthma attack so that you may take practical steps towards avoiding the irritant substance whenever possible.

THE HOUSE DUST MITE

The house dust mite, or to give it its proper name, *Dermatophagoides pteronnysinus* (from the Greek words meaning skin-eating feather mite), is the source of the major allergen causing asthma in the UK. It is one of almost 50 species of mites and has adapted very successfully to life in our homes. It is essentially a bed mite, since it feeds on human skin scales that are shed into our bedding during sleep. There is no shortage of food since one person sheds 0.5–1 gram of scales each day, sufficient to feed thousands of mites for months. Since their diet of skin scales is essentially dry, mites need to obtain fluid from the air, and for this reason the humidity in the atmosphere is usually the decisive factor determining the size of the mite population. Conditions of approximately 80 per cent relative humidity and 25° centigrade of warmth form an ideal habitat for mites. In London, the average monthly humidity varies between about 73 per cent in June to about 86 per cent in December, and it is not surprising that levels of infestation in British homes are high. In mountainous areas, particularly above 1,400 metres, mites are found in very low numbers, probably as the result of the low humidity and low temperatures at altitude. Mites vary in numbers in dust collected from bed mattresses, but infestation can be as high as 5,000 mites per gram of dust.

The mites themselves are very small, approximately 0.3 millimetres in size, and are indistinguishable from specks of dust to the naked eye. Under the microscope they look pretty unprepossessing. Despite their small size intact house dust mites are far too large to inhale deep into the nose or lungs, and studies have shown that the allergen causing asthma is found in the droppings or faeces of the mite. The allergen itself is a protein excreted by the mite's gut that is used to digest the human skin scales that it has eaten.

These faecal pellets are approximately 20 micrometres in size, that is, 20,000ths of a millimetre. They can easily be breathed into the nose causing perennial rhinitis, and fragments are easily inhaled into the lungs to cause the allergic reaction that leads to asthma. The chemical nature of the house dust mite allergen has been fully worked out and is called Der p1.

After bedrooms, house dust mites are found in greatest numbers in living rooms. Carpets and upholstered furniture can develop high mite counts in excess of 1,000 mites per gram of dust and extremely high levels of the mite allergen. You inhale mite allergens when dusting or vacuuming, and during the night from bedding as you continually move around while sleeping. During his or her first year of life, a baby who is born with an inherited predisposition to allergy can become sensitised to the house dust mite if exposed to 100 mites per gram of dust from mattresses and carpets. Severe attacks can be triggered at levels of 500 mites per gram of dust.

BECOMING SENSITISED
Try to keep the bedding of young babies and children as free from house dust mite as possible, particularly if asthma runs in your family. Early exposure may cause your child to become sensitised.

PETS

Pets are now one of the major causes of allergic disease, second only to the house dust mite, with up to 40 per cent of asthmatic children sensitised to the allergens of cats and/or dogs. It is not necessary to be in direct contact with a cat or dog for an attack of asthma to occur. Animal allergens are present in the air and dust in the home, and allergy sufferers can develop asthma as soon as they go into a home with a pet. The allergens themselves are found in dander (skin scales), hair, saliva and urine, and get everywhere in the home where the animal lives. Cat allergens are found mainly in the saliva, the sweat ducts and the tear ducts. The fur becomes coated with the allergen during grooming. Cat fur itself is not intrinsically allergenic. A cat can shed 0.2 grams of hair and dander each day, leading to high concentrations of this potent allergen in the house.

Dog allergen in the home comes mainly from dander, hair and saliva. Quite often an asthma sufferer will have problems with some breeds but not others. There is some suggestion that the offending allergen is the same in all breeds, and it is just the concentration that varies.

Rabbits, small rodents and caged birds are very popular pets. Rabbits and guinea pigs are usually housed outdoors, whereas gerbils, hamsters, mice, rats and birds are more likely to be kept in the living room or even in the bedroom. These creatures, especially budgies and hamsters, are particularly associated with allergic asthma. In small mammals, urine is the most potent source of allergen, and materials lining cages can be heavily contaminated. Allergens are released into the air as the animal moves round the cage, disturbing the lining.

MOULDS

In addition to *Alternaria*, which can cause asthma in the autumn, the spores from *Aspergillus fumigatus* are an important cause of severe asthma. *Aspergillus fumigatus* is widely distributed and often found in rotting vegetation.

ANIMALS AND ASTHMA
Family pets, especially hamsters, cats and dogs, are now a very common cause of allergy in children.

OCCUPATIONAL ALLERGENS

Reactive chemicals and allergens encountered in the workplace are an important cause of asthma, particularly in adults who also smoke. It is very important to recognise the possibility that dusts, vapours or fumes that you encounter at work may be the cause of your asthma, since avoiding the sensitising agent may get rid of it completely. On the other hand, if you are constantly exposed to the allergen over a long period of time, your symptoms may persist and even become permanent.

The commonest cause of occupational asthma is contact with the chemical toluene diisocyanate used in varnishes and paints. Soldering fluxes used in the electronics industry, and platinum salts encountered in

10 Steps to Mimimise Exposure to Allergens

There are many practical ways in which you can reduce your exposure to suspect allergens. Reduced exposure will mimimise the frequency and severity of your asthma attacks.

STEP 1   Reduce moisture and damp. Open a window or door to ventilate your bathroom and kitchen during and immediately after cooking, washing and bathing. To avoid moisture spreading to the rest of the house, keep the internal doors closed. Do not dry clothes indoors unless dryers are vented to the outside. Air bedding before making beds and maintain a background ventilation in bedrooms by keeping a window open whenever possible.

STEP 2   Prevent build-up of dust. Reduce the number of exposed surfaces on which dust builds up, especially if they are difficult to clean. Clean surfaces with a damp cloth. Vacuum clean soft furnishings and curtains, as well as carpets and floors with a properly maintained cleaner. Vacuum clean mattresses fortnightly. Replace pillows and buy new ones every three months if you can.

STEP 3   Wash bed linen at a high temperature (at least 60°C) to kill the house dust mite.

STEP 4   Enclose bedding and wash soft toys. Encase all mattresses, duvets and pillows in the sufferer's bedroom with microporous membrane covers. Many different types are now available and the costs vary. These covers need to be wiped clean with a damp cloth and completely dried each time you change the bed. Soft toys can contain large numbers of house dust mites, so choose ones that can be washed at 60°C and other toys that can be wiped down. Keep soft toys out of your child's bed.

STEP 5   Get rid of carpets. Wherever possible replace them with linoleum or vinyl flooring, or sealed natural flooring such as cork tiles or wood, with as few dust-retaining crevices as possible.

10 Steps to Mimimise Exposure to Allergens (cont'd)

STEP 6   When replacing your old vacuum cleaner with a new one, choose a
model that has a high efficiency filter – look for the "Allergy Friendly"
logo of the British Allergy Foundation.

STEP 7   Replace furnishings. Get rid of woven fabric-covered chairs or sofas and
opt instead for cane, canvas, leather or leather-like covered furnishings,
which are easy to clean and do not harbour house dust mites.

STEP 8   Change your home environment. Although not yet proven, it is likely that
a different type of heating system with improved through drafts will
reduce humidity and house dust mite numbers. Air filtration, dehumidifiers
and mechanical ventilation with heat recovery are all being tried. The
National Asthma Campaign, working with a building company, has created
the first low-allergen house, which embodies these steps to reduce
exposure to allergens. This approach is a step in the right direction for the
millions of sufferers of house dust mite allergy.

STEP 9   If at all possible, find a new home for your cat and/or dog. Giving your pet
frequent baths can be effective. Bathing a cat once a week can reduce the
allergens in the home by 90 per cent. Confining a cat to one part of the
house is unlikely to be effective, as people transfer cat allergens on their
clothes. Sadly, in allergic families, pets need to be banned. Even after the
animal has gone, it can be many months before the allergen levels in the
dust fall, and allergens can only be eliminated completely by replacement
of all floor coverings and upholstery, and by thorough cleaning.

STEP 10   Reduce humidity and dampness in your home. This will effectively prevent
the growth of the moulds that can cause asthma and other allergies.
Awareness and recognition of occupational causes of asthma can lead to
effective industrial hygiene, eliminating the problem altogether.

metal refining, are also important causes. Bakers can become allergic to flour, and farmers and dock workers allergic to grain, and indeed to the grain mite that flourishes in grain with a high water content. Carpenters and sawmill workers can become allergic to dusts from wood, and those working in the pharmaceutical industry to a number of the medicines manufactured. Increased recognition of this problem, as well as considerable improvements in ventilation and hygiene, should reduce the number of sufferers from occupational asthma.

The characteristic feature, which tends to confirm the diagnosis of occupational asthma, is that symptoms occur soon after starting the working day, but improve at weekends and may disappear on holidays.

AIR POLLUTION

There is no doubt many people suffer attacks of breathlessness and coughing – whether they have asthma or not – during episodes of air pollution caused by emissions from petrol and diesel engines and from the burning of coal and gas in power stations. When you do have asthma, the effects of pollution reduce the amount of allergen needed to bring on an attack. Moreover, pollution may bring on attacks of asthma in people who had previously only suffered from allergic rhinitis.

The cocktail of pollutant gases, sulphur dioxide, ozone and the oxides of nitrogen, together with small particulates, less than 10 micrometres in diameter, emitted from diesel engines (PM10s) may be particularly dangerous and lead directly to the deaths of people with severe asthma and other respiratory diseases. Whether pollutant gases are an important contributing factor to the increase in asthma remains to be determined.

OTHER TRIGGERS

Viral infections, particularly the common cold virus (known as the rhinovirus), readily trigger attacks of asthma, often followed by a prolonged period of coughing. If you have asthma, it is worth doing all you can to avoid contact with cold sufferers and be ready to double the dose of treatment you are taking to control your symptoms. Like people with allergic rhinitis, you may be one of the one in 20 asthma sufferers who have a severe attack after taking aspirin or other non-steroidal anti-inflammatory drugs such as ibuprofen (Nurofen). Of additional concern to asthma sufferers, is the use of tablets used to treat high blood pressure. You should never take one frequently prescribed type of treatment known as the beta-blockers, since they block the beneficial effect of the naturally occurring adrenaline in the blood, which helps to keep the airways of the lung open. There have been deaths among asthma sufferers who have been prescribed these drugs.

HOW IS IT TREATED?

At the present time there are no medicines that can cure asthma. For this reason it is essential to try to minimise exposure to the important allergens that can initially sensitise babies in the first year of life, and subsequently cause attacks of asthma. This can be done in a step-by-step approach (see pp.52–53).

PLANNING TREATMENT

The doctors who are managing your asthma will have specific goals in mind

The Aims of Asthma Treatment Targets

Any programme of asthma treatment should aim to ensure that:

- You lead a full, active life.
- You keep your lung function as near to normal as possible.
- You are able to take part in sporting activity if you want to – whether you are an adult or a child.
- You lose no time from school or work.
- You suffer no night-time symptoms.

The Five Treatment Steps for Asthma

There are many drugs that can be used to treat asthma. However, since the symptoms and severity of an attack vary enormously, treatment must be tailored to the needs of the individual.

STEP 1

Occasional use of a bronchodilator inhaler, such as salbutamol (Ventolin) or terbutaline (Bricanyl). Using this treatment by itself is only recommended if your asthma is very infrequent and your lung function normal.

STEP 2

Regular anti-allergic treatment with sodium cromoglycate (Intal) or nedocromil sodium (Tilade). This treatment, taken regularly, is the best therapy if your asthma attacks occur on a regular basis and your lung function, as measured by a peak flow meter, is essentially normal. The anti-leukotriene drug Singulair which is taken as one tablet at night is also effective.

STEP 3

Anti-inflammatory treatment with beclomethasone dipropionate (Becotide) or budesonide (Pulmicort) inhalers. These corticosteroid inhalers are extremely effective, when taken regularly, in controlling asthma symptoms and improving lung function, and should be used if anti-allergic treatment is not keeping your asthma under control and your lung function normal.

When beclomethasone dipropionate (Becotide) or budesonide (Pulmicort) are used at doses ranging from 100–800 micrograms per day, side-effects are rarely a problem.

Occasionally, deposition of the aerosol spray at the back of the throat leads to a yeast infection known as candidiasis (thrush). This may cause a sore throat and sometimes weakening of the voice. Brushing your teeth, gargling or eating immediately after using the inhalers is the best way to prevent any of the corticosteroid spray remaining at the back of your throat.

The Five Treatment Steps (cont'd)

STEP 4

High-dose anti-inflammatory treatment with budesonide (Pulmicort) at a dose of 1600 micrograms per day, or fluticasone propionate (Flixotide) at a dose of 1-2 mg per day. The use of higher doses of inhaled corticosteroids may be required if your asthma is not controlled using the lower doses, or during a bad phase caused, for example, by pollution or the common cold virus.

At higher doses these corticosteroids are absorbed into the bloodstream to a significant extent and may be associated with some side-effects. Remember to reduce the dose once your symptoms are under control and your lung function improved.

STEP 5

Tablets of the corticosteroid, prednisolone. This is an emergency treatment for severe attacks of asthma. Tablets of prednisolone taken at high doses above 15 mg per day for long periods of time will be associated with the development of side-effects. These include indigestion, thinning and bruising of the skin, wasting of muscles and thinning of the bones. A short course of prednisolone over a few weeks, however, is highly unlikely to be associated with such side-effects and may be necessary to relieve severe symptoms and improve reduced lung function.

when choosing the right treatment for you. The emphasis has moved away from treatment of asthma symptoms as they arise and towards giving sufficient anti-allergic and anti-inflammatory treatment to prevent symptoms occurring in the first place. This has led to the development of a step-by-step plan (set out on pp.56–57) for the management of asthma with the aim of preventing symptoms and keeping lung function, as measured by the peak-flow meter, as near normal as is possible. Should peak flows fall by 20 per cent from your best recorded measurements, you will need higher doses of anti-allergic and anti-inflammatory treatment. It is vital that you are able to inhale your asthma medications effectively. The advantage of taking medicines in this way is that the amount absorbed into the bloodstream is very low and side-effects are largely avoided.

ANTI-INFLAMMATORIES
Some drugs, such as these anti-inflammatories, may precipitate a severe asthma attack in certain susceptible individuals.

HOW TO USE AN INHALER

It's not always easy to acquire the knack of inhaling the spray from a metered dose inhaler. You have to breathe in at the same time as activating the inhaler to release the correct dose. Some people never manage this technique effectively, but there are many devices available to help. The medicine can be initially sprayed into and then breathed out of a spacer device, so you do not have to synchronise triggering the inhaler and breathing in. Devices that contain the asthma medication in the form of a dry powder are easier to use since after loading the inhaler, all you have to do is simply breathe the powder into your lungs. Such devices include spinhalers, diskhalers and turbohalers. Make sure you use the inhaler device that you find suits you best. As yet, none of the medicines needed for the treatment of asthma is available without prescription.

You can use bronchodilator treatment whenever you need it at any step in the treatment of asthma, but remember that if you have to use your inhaler more than four times a day, it is best to increase the dose of anti-allergic and anti-inflammatory treatment.

Barrel

Mouthpiece

Capsule

INTAL SPINHALER
The inhaled drug sodium cromoglycate can be taken using a delivery device such as this Intal spinhaler. The capsules contain the drug in a powder form, which is breathed into the lungs.

KEY POINTS

- Asthma is becoming more common in developed countries.
- The symptoms of asthma include breathlessness, wheezing, chest tightness and coughing.
- Common triggers of asthma attacks include the house dust mite, family pets and moulds.
- It is important to limit exposure to known allergens whenever possible.
- There are a number of drugs that can prevent and treat asthma.

Peanut and other food allergies

Reactions to foods are extremely common, although only a very small proportion of the symptoms that develop after eating particular foods are true allergies, meaning that they involve the body's immune system.

FOOD AVERSION
A child's refusal to eat certain foods is more often the result of a dislike than an allergy, but serious aversions should nontheless be investigated.

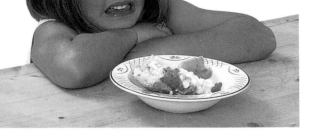

Everyone has their likes and dislikes when it comes to food, and young children often refuse particular foods as part of their drive for independence. However, in later life over-eating or rejection of certain foods (food faddism) is usually the result of psychological factors, which are not clearly understood.

The most severe form of food aversion is anorexia nervosa, characterised by a determined refusal to eat. This eating disorder usually begins in adolescence. Anorexics, who can be very manipulative, often persuade their carers that they have severe food allergies causing a wide range of symptoms. In this way they may be able to disguise the anorexia and become classified as suffering from the total allergy syndrome. Apart from aversion, other reactions to foods are best described as food intolerances. Food intolerance encompasses normal reactions to large amounts of specific foods, the irritant effects of foods, results of deficiency in the enzymes necessary to break up foods and true food allergy.

— NORMAL REACTIONS TO FOOD —

Caffeine is the most popular and widely used stimulant drug in the world, and it produces side-effects at doses of only 200 milligrams – just two moderately strong cups of coffee. It is addictive and particularly affects the nerves, heart and stomach. Too much coffee and your hands shake, your heart races, your oesophagus (the food-pipe) relaxes, causing subsequent heartburn, and your sleep is disturbed. Some types of cheeses and pickled fish contain tyramine, chocolate contains phenylethylamine and citrus fruits, octopamine. Bananas, avocados, yeast extract and wine contain similar compounds that can affect and cause widening of the blood vessels, bringing on migraine in susceptible people, flushing of the face and the widespread itchy skin eruption known as nettle rash or urticaria.

Histamine is found in some cheeses, sauerkraut and sausages such as pepperoni and salami. Bacteria can produce histamine, and high levels of this potent chemical can be found in fish, particularly mackerel that has been kept too long. Consuming large amounts of histamine causes urticaria, swelling of the lips, face and tongue, and intense headaches.

FOODS TO AVOID
Cheese contains tyramine, a substance that can trigger headaches or migraine in susceptible people.

IRRITANT EFFECTS OF FOOD

Stomach ache, wind, constipation and diarrhoea are extremely common, affecting almost everyone. The food we eat influences symptoms, altering the tenderness of the gut, production of gas and composition of the faeces – a well-known example being curry powder.

The persistence of such symptoms without any serious underlying cause is called irritable bowel syndrome, which is very common and as yet poorly understood. Nevertheless avoiding foods which exacerbate symptoms, increasing the amount of fibre in the diet and learning to cope better with stress can all be helpful.

ENZYME DEFICIENCIES

Low levels of an enzyme called lactase, which breaks down milk, is a rare but important cause of severe watery diarrhoea in children, when they are fed cow's milk. In some ethnic groups, for example among Chinese people, where milk plays little part in the diet, levels of lactase are extremely low and drinking milk or eating milk products leads to diarrhoea.

Lactase levels may be temporarily reduced by many common bowel disorders such as gastroenteritis, and drinking milk can cause diarrhoea for many months following the illness, so it's best to avoid milk until the enzymes return to their normal level.

Alcohol, too, can cause problems for particular groups of people. Alcohol is broken down in the body by a series of enzymes, one of which is called aldehyde dehydrogenase. Up to 40 per cent of Japanese people have very low levels of this enzyme and are therefore particularly susceptible to the effects of drinking alcohol, which they learn to avoid.

FOOD ALLERGIES

Fifteen per cent of the population say that they suffer symptoms related to eating certain foods. It is possible to test this by disguising the food in a specially prepared meal and comparing the effects with the same meal not containing the suspected food allergen. This type of 'blinded food challenge' shows that the true frequency of allergies and intolerances occurs in less than two per cent of people. Nevertheless, allergy to milk, eggs, fish and nuts in particular can cause severe symptoms, particularly in children, and allergy to peanuts appears to be increasing at an alarming rate.

The symptoms that develop following contact with a minute amount of the food are well recognised. In highly allergic sufferers, mere contact between the offending food and the lips causes tingling and rapid swelling of the lips within seconds to minutes. This is followed by swelling of the tongue which if severe enough can cause obstruction at the back of the mouth and suffocation unless the appropriate treatment, in the form of an injection of adrenaline, is rapidly given. If the food has been eaten, the person vomits violently and severely, and if some of the food allergen has been absorbed into the bloodstream they develop a widespread urticarial rash, start to wheeze and their blood pressure drops steeply.

ANAPHYLACTIC SHOCK
Rarely, food allergies can be life-threatening. Contact with the offending food can cause a severe reaction, with collapse and difficulty in breathing.

This generalised reaction is called anaphylaxis, and without treatment, it can and does lead to tragic loss of life. Sometimes the onset of food- allergic symptoms can be more insidious and difficult to diagnose, requiring the expert help of a dietician. In this case, the sufferer will be involved in careful research, recording what foods they've eaten over the preceding weeks in a diary, which can then be studied in relation to their symptoms.

One way of confirming the diagnosis is to put the sufferer on a strict elimination diet that includes a very restricted number of foods: for example, one meat, one fruit, one vegetable, one starch source. The choice of foods is based on those least likely to cause allergic reactions, such as lamb or chicken, rhubarb or pears, carrots or sprouts, and rice or potato. A fat source, such as a milk-free margarine or specific vegetable oil, and sugar may also be allowed. If symptoms settle on this strict elimination diet additional foods can then be added, and if symptoms develop the source of the problem is easily identified.

One of the most difficult problems you'll encounter if you have a food allergy is how to know whether prepared foods contain the offending allergen. A good example is allergy to peanuts.

PEANUT ALLERGY

The peanut is actually related to the pea and is a legume, not a nut. Like other peas it bears its fruit in pods (shells), but the unusual thing is that they develop underground. Between 15 million and 18 million metric tons of peanuts are harvested every year, especially in Asia, Africa and the United States. For anyone who's not allergic to them, they are a very healthy food: there is more protein in peanuts than in the equivalent weight of beefsteak. As well as being a food in itself, the peanut is a greater source of edible oil than almost any other commercially grown crop. Peanuts are passed through rollers, which grind them

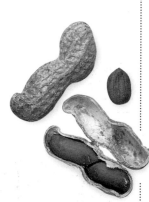

THE HIDDEN INGREDIENT
Whole peanuts are easy to detect and avoid, but peanut oil is a hidden ingredient in many food products.

into small particles, and then squeezed through a press. Alternatively, a chemical solvent is used to dissolve the oil. It's known that, unless specially prepared, peanut oil still contains the peanut allergen, and peanut oil is widely used in prepared foods, both as the oil itself and as a carrier for fat-soluble vitamins and colourings.

Apart from foods the uses of peanuts are many and various. Low-grade oil is used as an ingredient in soaps, shaving creams, shampoos and even paints, and in the manufacture of the explosive nitroglycerine. Peanut oil, listed as arachis oil, is a component of some medicinal products including skin care products which might be prescribed for allergic patients.

Many children with extreme peanut allergy have never been knowingly exposed to peanuts prior to their first reaction, raising the question of how they became sensitised. Peanut oil was a common constituent of many infant milk formulas, but there is now no peanut oil in Cow & Gate infant milk formulas, Heinz infant milk formula, Milupa, Sainsbury's infant milk formula or in SMA infant milk formulas.

Another concern is that there may be cross-reactivity between peanuts and soya, which is a common constituent of infant milk formulas. Research into this is urgently required.

INFANT MILK FORMULAS
Although most manufacturers have now discontinued the use of peanut oil in infant milk formulas, parents should check the ingredients of all baby foods.

FOOD-ADDITIVE ALLERGIES

A food additive is any substance not commonly used as a food but which is added to a food at any stage to affect its keeping quality, texture, consistency, taste or smell. Food additives may trigger urticaria, asthma and rhinitis, and the most important food colouring that is known to cause symptoms is the yellow dye tartrazine (E102), which is frequently added to many pre-packaged convenience foods. In addition, tartrazine is usually present in smoked cod and haddock, lime and lemon squash, salad cream and marzipan, and, somewhat surprisingly, in mint sauce and jelly, brown sauce and tinned processed peas.

Another yellow colouring, sunset yellow (E110), is present in orange squash, fish fingers, lemon curd and Lucozade. Benzoates (E211) are preservatives, preventing the growth of bacteria and fungi, and they are added to many drinks, for example soft drinks, squashes and beer, and also to margarine.

The number of people who suffer from reactions to food additives is relatively small, possibly making up only a tenth of those who suffer food intolerances. Nevertheless, food additives do pose a real problem, and one which is being taken increasingly seriously by food manufacturers. Thanks to improvement in labelling it is increasingly possible to identify which foods contain the chemicals that provoke symptoms for you and so avoid consuming them.

DIAGNOSIS OF FOOD ALLERGIES

Skin testing and blood tests (CAP-RAST) can be very helpful in identifying a food allergy to milk, egg, fish, shellfish, wheat, soya, peanuts and true nuts. However, blinded food challenges and strict elimination diets, which should be followed only under proper medical supervision, may be necessary in the diagnosis of more complex cases.

The European Food Intolerance Databank

This data bank is designed to provide up-to-date information about food products and their ingredients for people who suffer from particular food intolerances and allergies.

A joint initiative between the British Dietetic Association, the Food and Drink Federation and the Leatherhead Food Research Association led to the development of a database in the UK, and now in Europe, containing details of ingredients and additives.

The databank can be accessed by your dietitian. Information from food retailers and manufacturers is carefully checked and covers the following food additives and ingredients:

- Sulphur dioxide ● Benzoate ● Glutamate ● Azo-colours
- Milk ● Egg ● Wheat ● Soya ● Derivatives of these ingredients

Many supermarket chains now have detailed lists of all the constituents of their prepared foods and some, together with the British Allergy Foundation, have prepared leaflets covering the main food allergies.

TREATMENT OF FOOD ALLERGIES

If you suffer from a food allergy, the most effective form of treatment is to cut the offending food out of your diet. To ensure that your diet remains nutritionally adequate, you should consult a professional dietician. Mild reactions to a food allergy can be treated with antihistamines, but more severe and life-threatening reactions must be treated with adrenaline.

DIET

Cutting out the food which is causing your intolerance or allergy is the key to successful treatment. However, it is vital that you make sure that your diet is nutritionally adequate, providing sufficient protein, energy, vitamins and minerals, particularly calcium. This is especially important in young children whose growth rate can be impaired by poorly designed low-energy elimination diets. Do not adopt a very restrictive diet without professional help from a dietician.

ANTIHISTAMINES

Antihistamines are useful for the treatment of the milder manifestations of food allergy, where the symptoms are confined to itching and swelling of the lips, swelling of the face (angio-oedema) and urticaria. Loratadine (Clarityn) or cetirizine (Zirtek) are the antihistamines you should opt for. They are, however, of no value in the event of more severe life-threatening reactions, including swelling of the tongue, asthma and falling blood pressure.

EPI-PENS AND MIN-I-JETS

The only effective treatment for the severe food allergies causing life-threatening reactions is adrenaline. This medicine will cause constriction of the blood vessels in the swollen lips, face and tongue, reverse the asthma and raise blood pressure. It must be administered rapidly. Treating severe allergic reactions to foods yourself has been revolutionised by the introduction of the Epi-pen auto-injector. This has a spring-activated concealed needle and is designed to deliver a single 0.3 milligram dose of adrenaline into a muscle when the pen is pushed firmly against the outer thigh. The children's version contains 0.15 milligrams of adrenaline. Min-i-jet adrenaline is an alternative but this consists of a 1 millilitre disposable syringe and needle, and you have to

Tube containing adrenaline dose

Safety cap covering needle

THE EPI-PEN
A measured dose of adrenaline can be self-administered quickly and easily with an Epi-pen.

measure the dose needed since a full syringe will deliver 1 milligram of adrenaline. Most people much prefer the Epi-pen which is easy to use, has no needle visible and has a shelf-life of two years compared to the nine months of the Min-i-jet adrenaline.

While the Min-i-jet adrenaline may contain too large a dose of adrenaline, the Epi-pen auto-injector may not give a big enough dose to treat severe anaphylactic reactions. For this reason you should always carry two Epi-pens with you, so that you can use the second one 10 minutes after the first if your symptoms are not responding adequately.

If you are at risk from severe allergic reactions, you must carry the Epi-pens with you wherever you go. When the sufferer is a child, it may be best to have Epi-pens at home and at school. Increasingly, teachers are prepared to administer adrenaline, particularly using the Epi-pen, once they have had advice and training. Because of the increasing frequency of peanut allergy, some schools are becoming nut-free zones.

MEDIC-ALERT AND ALLERGY PATCHES

If you have a life-threatening allergy, you must make this fact known so that appropriate treatment can be given if you are unconscious when emergency medical treatment arrives. Medic-Alert provides a bracelet or necklet containing medical details and a 24-hour emergency number. For further details, call free on 0800 581420. Allergy patches with the words 'I am allergic to nuts', for example, can be helpful in young children at nursery or primary school. Fixed on to outer clothing, allergy patches immediately highlight the sufferer's problem to teachers and other children and parents.

KEY POINTS

- True food allergies – those that involve the body's immune system – are extremely rare.
- Reactions to food may be caused by a lack of a particular digestive enzyme.
- Food allergy can cause severe symptoms including swelling of the lips and tongue, wheezing and low blood pressure.
- The best treatment for food allergy is to cut the offending food from the diet.
- Severe reactions must be treated with adrenaline.

Itchy skin rashes

Itchy skin disorders may be caused by an allergy to certain substances that come into contact with the skin. The skin becomes inflamed and itchy, and there may also be blistering. Many substances are known to precipitate an attack, including certain foods, plants and cosmetics.

URTICARIA

Urticaria closely resembles the itchy white blisters and red patches that result from nettle stings, and the reaction in the skin is mainly due to histamine from mast cells. The symptoms can occur on any part of your body, and normally come and go over the space of a few hours. Acute, short-lasting attacks of urticaria are very common, affecting as many as one in five of the population at some stage in their lives.

Anyone who is allergic to dogs, for example, will rapidly develop a red itchy rash when licked on the face by a dog. Food allergy sufferers frequently develop swelling of the lips or inside of the mouth after eating eggs, milk or nuts. Sometimes this type of contact urticaria can be triggered by intolerances to chemicals including ammonia, bleaches and preservatives, as well as to nettles and the primula plant. When you eat something you're allergic to, you'll get widespread urticarial

DOGS AND ALLERGIES
Even pet owners can find that they react to close contact with their animal's fur or saliva.

71

rashes all over your body. Well-known causes – in addition to milk, egg and nuts – are fish, shellfish, beans, potatoes, strawberries, celery, parsley and spices. You'll get this type of rash following a bee or wasp sting if you're allergic to the venom of these insects, and many medicines, particularly penicillin, are associated with widespread itchy rashes.

If no external cause for the urticaria can be found and the skin rash persists over several weeks, then other causes will need to be identified.

Some people find that changes in temperature and pressure can bring on the rash, and in children with this condition a hereditary absence of a blocking protein in the blood may be the cause, particularly if other members of the family are similarly affected. In severe and long-lasting urticaria the body may be reacting against itself with the development of an antibody against the mast cell which causes it to release histamine. You may be one of the many urticaria sufferers who knows the cause of your skin rash so that you can avoid the triggering food. In other people skin prick testing or RAST may help to discover the offending allergen. Elimination diets may help. Antihistamines are particularly helpful in blocking the effect of histamine released from mast cells in the skin which causes this itchy rash. Taking a non-sedating antihistamine such as cetirizine or loratadine once a day will relieve the symptoms rapidly and effectively.

However, finding a permanent cure for the problem means identifying the cause whenever possible and avoiding the allergen once you know what it is.

STRAWBERRIES
These seemingly innocuous fruits are one of the most common causes of an allergic reaction to food and can cause an itchy rash to appear all over the body.

SKIN SWELLINGS

Angio-oedema simply means a deep swelling in the tissues, particularly of the face, tongue and larynx, caused by the effects of histamine and other chemicals released from mast cells which cause the blood vessels to leak fluid into the tissues. It is closely linked to urticaria with similar causes and like urticaria can be triggered by both allergens and intolerance to a number of medicines as well as preservatives. The commonest triggering factor in up to 75 per cent of sufferers is aspirin and the closely related non-steroidal anti-inflammatory drugs such as ibuprofen (Nurofen). Occasionally paracetamol can be the cause. Preservatives and colourings also need to be avoided, particularly benzoic acid, ascorbic acid, parabens, sulphites and anti-oxidants. One particular type of modern medicine used to treat raised blood pressure and heart failure, known as the angiotensin-converting enzyme inhibitors or ACE inhibitors, can cause severe urticaria and angio-oedema. Swelling of the tongue and larynx causes increasing breathlessness and can be fatal unless rapidly treated by injection of adrenaline.

ITCHY CRACKED SKIN

The commonest causes of itchy, scaly, weepy red rash are atopic eczema and contact dermatitis.

ATOPIC ECZEMA

This rash starts between the ages of two and six months, often on the face, and the irritation keeps the baby awake. The rash can spread over the body, but the nappy area is not involved. In about half of the children affected in this way, the rash clears by 18 months of age. In the remainder the rash moves to the skin folds, particularly the inside of

Common Eczema Sites on Children

Eczema, which causes itchy, scaly, reddened skin,
can occur on any part of the body, but in young children
this condition commonly affects particular areas.

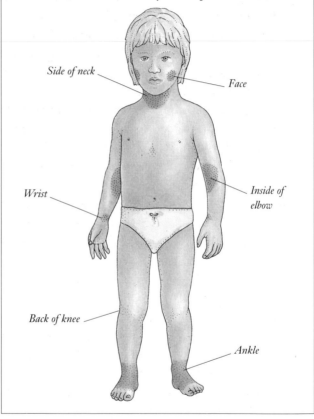

Side of neck

Face

Wrist

Inside of
elbow

Back of knee

Ankle

the elbows and the backs of the knees. Additionally the skin on the side of the neck, wrists and ankles is affected, and in toddlers eczema often persists on the face.

Atopic eczema is less common in adults. The rash principally affects skin folds where thickening can occur.

Emotional problems can prolong the course of the disease but it usually disappears on its own by the age of 30. Localised patches of eczema can occur on the lips and sometimes on the nipples in young women. Eczema may reappear on parts of the body which are under physical stress for some reason – for example, on the hands of nurses and hairdressers. Eczema affecting the hands and feet often appears as small blisters under the skin and in older people patches of eczema are often associated with varicose veins around the ankles.

The part played by allergy to house dust mite, pets and foods in causing atopic eczema remains controversial. However, the National Child Development Study has shown that eczema recorded by physical examination is almost twice as common in better off people as compared to those with lower incomes. This finding indicates that environmental exposure and lifestyle are at least as important as genetic factors in the development of childhood eczema.

Factors which might explain this difference include the amount of carpets and central heating in the home (because of their influence on the house dust mite population), use of showers and soaps, exposure to ultraviolet light, contact with pets, age of the mother and diet. Seventy five per cent of children with severe atopic eczema have very high concentrations of IgE antibody to the mite allergen, and patch tests with mite allergens produce a positive result. The application of mite allergen to eczematous skin makes the rash worse, and children improve in hospital where mite counts are low, even when they're being given no specific treatment.

Some sufferers notice the development of eczema around their eyes and nose during the pollen season, adding further misery to their allergic conjunctivitis and rhinitis. Twenty five per cent of eczema sufferers are allergic to eggs, milk, nuts, wheat, fish and shellfish. Apart from the development of contact urticaria around the face and mouth on contact with food, sufferers describe itching and worsening of eczema eight to 24 hours later. Eczema often starts after babies are weaned from breast milk, and giving them formula milk instead of cows' milk can sometimes cause a dramatic improvement. Similarly, reducing a child's exposure to house dust mite and pets can be helpful. It is possible to at least delay the onset of infant eczema, in at risk babies born to allergic parents by breast feeding as long as possible, avoiding cows' milk, taking house dust mite control measures, banishing pets and banning smoking in the home.

The basic treatment for eczema is use of emollients and avoiding the use of soap. Sufferers often find that one of the many available emollients suits them better than the others, and this should be applied regularly throughout the day and particularly after a bath or shower. If avoiding allergens and using emollients doesn't solve the problem, corticosteroid ointments and creams are the best form of treatment. The key principle is to use the least potent steroid preparation needed to keep eczema under control and when possible stop the treatment for short periods. For many children one per cent cortisone ointment is adequate. Potent steroid creams and ointments should be used with caution for limited periods only.

Some patients have benefited considerably from using evening primrose oil (Epogam) at appropriate doses of 160–320 milligrams daily in children and 320–480 milligrams in adults. It's worth trying it for three months if other simpler measures have failed, but if there's no

Chinese Herbal Medicine

There are many hundreds of clinics offering traditional Chinese medicines. These have produced impressive responses in cases of atopic eczema that have proved resistant to conventional medicine.

Usually Chinese herbal treatment involves drinking a tea prepared from 10 or so plant materials tailored to the individual patient. Although there is no doubt that some of the plant materials used by the Chinese for treating eczema are beneficial, and in some cases better than Western treatment, unfortunately the effect is usually temporary, with a relapse occurring after six to twelve months. In addition the herbal remedies may damage the liver. Careful analysis of the compounds present in the plant materials may in the future lead to better standardised, safer and more effective therapies for eczema.

Herbal infusion

Strainer

Chinese herbal tea

improvement within that time, it's not worth continuing. Antihistamines are of little benefit in the management of atopic eczema. Worsening eczema may be the result of secondary infection with bacteria requiring treatment with the appropriate antibiotic from the doctor.

ALLERGIC CONTACT DERMATITIS

Unlike allergic eczema this disease is more common with advancing age. Symptoms are redness, scaling and thickening of the skin, which itches where it has been in contact with the allergen – for example,

Common Allergens

Some individuals develop an allergic reaction to chemicals that are to be found in everyday substances such as cosmetics, bleaches and jewellery. The diagnosis can be confirmed by patch testing, and avoiding the allergen is the cure.

NICKEL
Clothing clasps, spectacle frames, jewellery, coins, household utensils

CHROMATE
Leather, bleaches, matches, cement

FORMALDEHYDE
Preservatives, cosmetics, nail varnish, newsprint, cigarettes, fabric conditioners, wrinkle-resistant clothes

ETHYLENE DIAMINE
Preservatives in creams, paints

MERCAPTOBENZOTHIAZOLE
Rubber products, especially boots, gloves and catheters

THIURAMS
Rubber products, fungicides in paint and soap

PLANTS
Primula, poison ivy, dahlias, chrysanthemums

on the face with cosmetics and aftershave, and on the ears from the nickel that is sometimes present in earrings. The hands are affected in two-thirds of contact dermatitis, much of which is due to contact with sensitising agents that have been encountered at work.

Many people who have skin conditions find that they're better when they've been out in the sun, but sunlight can itself cause a rash in fair-skinned people. The answer is to use a sunblock cream.

Some perfumes, cosmetics, eye lotions and even the sunscreen products themselves contain chemicals – usually preservatives and antiseptics – that increase the skin's sensitivity to sunlight, as can some antibiotics, leading to a red, itchy rash when you sunbathe.

An increasing and worrying problem is allergy to natural rubber latex used in balloons, condoms and particularly in gloves. One in 10 health care workers in the USA are now affected, with the proportion up to 17 per cent in one hospital. The allergy is increasing in Britain as more and more dentists, nurses and health care professionals wear gloves, not just when operating but when taking and handling blood and other body fluids. The reaction varies from allergic contact dermatitis on the hands due to chemicals used in the manufacturing process to urticaria on the hand associated with asthma, anaphylaxis and even death. People with this allergy must ensure that doctors and dentists treating them use non-latex gloves, by wearing a Medic-Alert bracelet or necklet, which could be life-saving.

HYPO-ALLERGENIC COSMETICS

Sixty per cent of women say they have a sensitive skin, and hypo-allergenic cosmetics are increasingly popular. Lanolin and particularly preservatives and perfumes are the common skin sensitisers. If you have sensitive or allergy-prone skin, it's best to choose cosmetics without perfume and those containing the minimum of pigments, since each carries its own risk of allergy. Check that products are in narrow-necked tubes or jars since they are less likely to be contaminated with bacteria and preservatives. 'Air-backless' tubes prevent air being sucked in and prevent contamination with bacteria. Don't use products after the expiry date.

KEY POINTS

- Urticaria is often triggered by a food allergy.
- Eczema among young children is very common.
- Allergic contact dermatitis becomes more common with advancing age.

- Widespread reactions require emergency treatment with adrenaline. Use the Epi-pen immediately if you have any difficulty breathing, you feel dizzy or if a rash appears away from the sting. Always carry two Epi-pens wherever you go all year round if you're allergic to bees, and in summer and autumn for wasp allergy.
- Hyposensitisation (specific allergen injection immunotherapy) is the best way to prevent widespread reactions and anaphylaxis to wasp and bee stings. Increasing concentrations and amounts of the venom are injected under the skin (subcutaneously) at weekly intervals for 15 weeks. The top dose, which is usually 100 micrograms of the venom, is then injected monthly for three years. This provides over 90 per cent protection which lasts for many years. The diagnosis of wasp and bee allergy and hyposensitisation treatment can only be provided in specialist hospital centres.

KEY POINTS

- Wasp and bee stings can cause large local reactions.
- Take preventive measures to avoid being stung.
- Treat stings with antihistamine or adrenaline.

Useful addresses

The Anaphylaxis Campaign
For information on peanut/
food anaphylaxis (that is to say,
immediate allergic reaction).
PO Box 149
Fleet
Hants GU13 9XU
Tel: (01252) 542029

**The British Allergy
Foundation (BAF)**
This organisation was founded
in June 1991 by a group of
leading medical specialists
determined to improve the
awareness, prevention and
treatment of allergy. The
British Allergy Foundation
encompasses all types of
allergy and aims to offer
information and support to
sufferers as well as raising
funds for allergy-related
research. Work is mainly
funded by voluntary income
and a small government
grant towards the cost of
the Allergy Helpline.
Deepdene House
30 Bellegrove Road
Welling, Kent DA16 3PY
Tel: (0181) 303 8525
Allergy Helpline:
Tel: (0189) 516 500

**The British Lung
Foundation**
This charity was established
in 1985 to raise funds for
research into all forms of lung
disease. They also have a
series of self-help groups
around the country, The
Breathe Easy Club, which
are largely run by patients.
78 Hatton Gardens
London EC1N 8LD
Tel: (0171) 831 5831
Fax: (0171) 831 5832

**Medic–Alert Foundation
For medical SOS necklets
& bracelets.**
1 Bridge Wharf
156 Caledonian Road
London N1 9UU
Tel: (0171) 833 3034
Freephone: 0800 581420

**Ministry of Agriculture,
Fisheries & Food**
Food Safety Directorate,
Chemical Safety of Food
Division.
For information on all foods.
Room 504A
Eron House
17 Smith Square
London SW1P 3JR
Tel: (0171) 238 6267

**National Asthma Campaign
(NAC)**
This is the only charity solely
dedicated to asthma. It raises
funds for research and is the
biggest contributor to asthma
research in the UK. It has an
active network of local groups
run by asthmatics for
asthmatics who provide a
variety of services to their
local population apart from
raising remarkable amounts
of money for research. It was
formed by the amalgamation
of the Asthma Society and the
Asthma Research Council.
Providence Place
London N1 0NT
Tel: (0171) 226 2260
Asthma Helpline:
(0345) 010203

**The National Eczema
Society**
163 Eversholt Street
London NW1 1BU
Tel: (0171) 388 4097

J. Sainsbury plc
For information & product
guides on dietary needs.
Stamford House, Stamford
Street, London SE1 9LL
Tel: (0171) 695 6000

Notes

Index

Acknowledgements

PUBLISHER'S ACKNOWLEDGEMENTS
Dorling Kindersley would like to thank the following for their help
and participation in this project:

Production Controller Michelle Thomas; **Consultancy** Dr. Sue Davidson;
Indexing Indexing Specialists, Hove; **Administration** Christopher Gordon.

Illustrations (p.14, p.24, p.28) Neal Johnson; (p.42, p.43) ©Philip Wilson

Picture Research Angela Anderson; **Picture Librarian** Charlotte Oster.

PICTURE CREDITS
The publisher would like to thank the following for their kind
permission to reproduce their photographs. Every effort has been made
to trace the copyright holders. Dorling Kindersley apologises for any
unintentional omissions and would be pleased, in any such cases,
to add an acknowledgement in future editions.

APM Studios p.21, p.47, p.58, p.59, p.68;
Oxford Scientific Films p.30 (GI Bernard), p.31 (John Brown);
Science Photo Library p.17 (Sheila Terry), p.33 (Keith Kent), p.39 (Geoff Tompkinson);
Telegraph Colour Library front cover, p.11 (L.Lefkowitz), p.60 (Robert Clare).

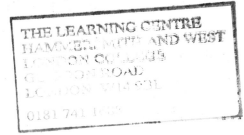